Green Smoothie
Cleanse

Delicious Weight   Loss Recipes

Steven Ballinger

Legal Disclaimer

Table of Contents

1: Just What is a Green Smoothie?

No, a green smoothie isn't a smoothie that is committed to driving hybrid vehicles. Instead, it's a fruit smoothie – but it is green. It gets its color from leafy, raw greens that go into the blending process. It still tastes like fruit, but it's green.

The cool thing about greens is that they are very nutritious; however, most people do not get enough of them in their diet – and flavor is often part of the problem. If you add fruit, you can make the greens taste better, and you're getting both fruit and vegetables in your daily nutrition.

A green smoothie is a terrific way to knock out both of those food groups.
There are many benefits from drinking green smoothies. Yes, you get more fruits and vegetables. However, you will also notice improvements in your digestion, clearer skin, a drop in weight and even a better mood.

People who follow the raw food diet have turned to green smoothies to give a boost to a diet that is already nutritious, and many find the vitality and sense of wellness that they want.

What do you put into a green smoothie?

It is important to emphasize that there are NO green smoothies that taste like spinach, asparagus, broccoli, Brussels sprouts or collard greens. Instead, they taste like their fruity ingredients. If you cram enough spinach into your smoothie, you will affect the flavor, but if you stick with the proportions from the recipes in this book, you will not taste the greens very much, if you taste them at all.

The majority of the green smoothies you will find in this book are primarily vegan and raw, which means that you won't find any dairy products, pasteurized ingredients or cooked substances. You won't find yogurt, sheep milk, goat milk, or cow milk, and you won't find soy, oat or rice milks. The alternatives to water are the plant based milks that come from seeds and nuts, for the most parts. There are some recipes that include honey and pollen, which are bee products, but you can substitute for those if you want to stay strictly vegan.

For the most part, a ratio of 60:40 between fruit and vegetables is what I recommend over time. To start with, you might start with 80:20 and even 90:10 until you get used to drinking your greens. If you find that your smoothie is a bit too green-tasting, add a dash of vanilla, sweetener or even a bit of lemon juice to get rid of that leafy flavor.

So how do you make a basic green smoothie?

The general formula is very simple. Add greens, some fruit and liquid into a blender and run it for a couple of minutes. You can put in the ingredients in any order. When the recipe suggests water, choose filtered or pure water. Always run the blender until you have a smooth texture.

Recipe for Your First Green Smoothie

Ingredients:
3 or 4 ripe bananas
2 cups water
1 teaspoon vanilla extract
Handful of clean, fresh raw spinach

Yield: About a liter

Basic Principles

You might think that combining a bunch of ingredients will give you a better smoothie. However, the simpler you keep things, the better the flavor will be. If you blend in five different fruits, you'll get a flavor that's fairly vague. If you blend bananas and strawberries in a smoothie, you'll generally get a good flavor that reveals both fruits. However, if you throw in plums, peaches and grapes, the smoothie won't really taste like any of the five fruits you've combined.

Choose fruits and vegetables that you already like to eat. If you don't, you are less likely to drink the smoothies that you make. It is possible to drink something that is great for you that is delicious at the same time. Part of the fun is inventing the smoothie that you really love. Sure, you're going to fail now and then and come up with a few things that your dog won't even sniff, but that's all right. Learning from those mistakes is what is important.

The most frequently used greens in my smoothie repertoire are spinach, parsley, Swiss chard, mint, kale and bok choy. A lot of green smoothie beginners like to use spinach, because it has a mild flavor and a brilliantly verdant color. Other vegetable influences that I will use include carrot tops, borage leaves, fennel tops, cilantro, radish tops, romaine, celery leaves, beet greens, basil, and parsley, as they all contribute to a successful green smoothie. If you are low on greens and run to the store for a bag salad, pick out those red leaves before you throw the salad mix in the blender. They tend to taste bitter, and so weeding them out can be quite helpful.

Make sure that you do not use the same greens each time you throw together a smoothie. Rotate your greens so that you always have something that is in season. You want to take in a diverse grouping of nutrients so that you are not always eating the same secondary metabolites (aka anti-nutrients).

One example is oxalic acid, which is found in spinach and Swiss chard. If you only use those two greens in all of your smoothies, you can develop a few problems. One issue is that oxalic acid will bind with calcium, meaning that your body will absorb less calcium from what you eat. A good rule of thumb is that you start to dread smoothies and feel ill in the middle of the morning, it's time for some new greens.

If you have your greens washed and ready for use, making smoothies doesn't take much time at all. What part of the greens should you use? Incorporate leaves from greens that have fibrous stalks (chard and kale are examples). Wash the leaves, and then set them out on dish towels to dry. Then, put another dry, clean towel on the bottom of a plastic container, and set the leaves in there to store in the refrigerator. The purpose of the towel is to absorb excess moisture, and you can leave the container in the refrigerator for five to seven days.

If you can, look for organic greens when you shop. They won't have herbicides or pesticides in their past, and they have more nutrients than greens grown using conventional methods. You can find a lot of these at farmer's markets if your local grocer does not carry organic greens.

If you have to settle for non-organic greens, make sure that you wash them thoroughly. If you have the time and room in your yard, it is easy to grow Swiss chard, even if you can't convince flowers to grow. It grows well in a yard garden or even in a pot on a balcony or courtyard.

2: So Why Are Greens So Important?

Greens have a huge amount of fiber, minerals, vitamins and antioxidants that are nutritionally crucial. They have fatty acids like the Omega-3s that are important for heart health. They don't have many calories, rate a low score on the glycemic index, don't have many carbs, have a lot of protein, and they are alkaline. They stimulate the activity of digestive enzymes and work to normalize your stomach acid levels.

One of the first proponents of the green smoothie was Victoria Boutenko, who believed that greens are the foods that come closest to completely meeting the nutritional needs that we have. The closest genetic relative to the human is the chimpanzee; we share more than 99 percent of the same parts of the genetic code.

The chimpanzee diet consists of about 50 percent fruits, 40 percent greens and 10 percent insects, bark and pith. The Western human diet, in contrast, consists of more than 50 percent cooked carbs, in the form of rice, pasta, bread and potatoes. About a third comes from animal protein, oils and fats, while the rest comes from vegetables and fruits.

Even in a best case scenario, the highest proportion that greens occupy in the Western diet is much smaller. Wild chimpanzees do not suffer from the same chronic ailments as their human counterparts, and the difference in consumption of greens could well be the reason behind the difference.

What's the deal with antioxidants, anyway?

Inside our body, exposure to toxins creates free radicals. These are molecules that have a single electron in the outer shell or layer. These are highly reactive molecules and will bond with something in order to gain stability. These will steal electrons from stable cells, in the process damaging cell structures like DNA, and by stealing electrons they create more free radicals. Antioxidants form the bonds that free radicals are missing without any damage happening to more molecules.

How do we digest greens?

Greens have internal cell walls that are made up of cellulose. For your body to gain access to the nutrients inside greens, those cell walls have to break. This means that we have to do a lot of chewing when we eat raw greens. However, we don't like to eat slowly, and our jaw muscles tire out fairly easily.

We also require strong acid in our stomachs to break down those walls, and not all of us have that. If you blend your greens to make a smoothie, the blender does that work for you, and you get the nutrients just from drinking. It is good to eat greens as well as drink green smoothies, but when you do eat greens, it is important to chew them thoroughly.

For people who are new to greens, they may only think that spinach and lettuce count. However, there are many more greens out there, and incorporating the whole spectrum ensures that you get the important nutrients from each one throughout your body.

If you're putting together a salad, there are many choices when it comes to greens: tatsoi, Swiss chard, spinach, sorrel, romaine, radicchio, oak leaf lettuce, mustard greens, mizuna, miner's lettuce, lamb's lettuce, kale, endive, dandelion greens, cress, cabbage, butter lettuce, bok choy, baby beet greens and arugula. Herbs like parsley, mint, cilantro and basil also work well frequently in salads.

The greens you should think about incorporating into your smoothies are similar to the ones that work well in salads. However, the more bitter greens, such as radicchio, and the ones with a hotter flavor, such as cress, mustard greens and arugula, will tend to overpower the fruit flavors in a smoothie. Instead, focus on greens within the cruciferous family, like kale and cabbage, when you start to make green smoothies. These have the antioxidants known as indoles as well as isothiocyanates, which are sulfur compounds that fight cancer.

Microgreens and sprouts are also used in both salads and smoothies, and they are extremely nutritious as well. You can even work in such common weeds from your backyard as dandelion, chickweed and parsley. Wild versions of endive, watercress, amaranth and alfalfa also are out there for you to try. Both of these types of greens are chock full of nutrients – often a great deal more so than their cultivated counterparts – and when you add variety to a diet, you keep things interesting in food preparation.

If you do want to try a wild food or weed, make sure that what you have gathered is not going to make you sick – or worse. Talk to a local expert who can show you indigenous plants. Those soft herbs that work well in salads can give your smoothie taste that is beyond special, and their nutritional properties do include a high level of antioxidants.

Is Juicing or Blending Better?

If you ask juicing and smoothie experts about this, each of them will talk about the great ways their own methods will help you. However, is one method better than the other? Those on the pro-juicing side argue that the fact that the juice has no fiber lets the concentrated nutrients go right into your bloodstream without a lot of digestive activity on your part. For those on the pro-smoothie side, it is the very presence of that fiber that makes that cool beverage such a great choice.

The function of the human digestive system is to break down foods so that the body can absorb them. However, when you drink juice, there is nothing to break down. You don't have to chew juice, and your digestive system expends almost no energy. Smoothies are simply juices with fiber blended inside; it is the very presence of that fiber that smoothie proponents indicate is their principal value.

So this means that a look at fiber is in order. Foods have two different sorts of fiber: soluble and insoluble. The body breaks down insoluble fiber during digestion, but it doesn't break it down all the way, and the smaller fragments go through the intestines molecularly intact, failing to contribute to nutrition or energy. The insoluble variety is present in high levels in leafy, green veggies. Soluble fiber, which you will find in foods like chia seeds and flax, turns into a gel in water and also zips along through your digestive tract without absorption.

So consider the consumption of orange through juicing, blending or eating. If you drink orange juice even with the pulp, you don't have to chew much and your stomach is the only part of the body that has to expend any energy.

The vitamins, antioxidants, minerals and sugars are all ready for your body to take in, and so they enter the bloodstream almost immediately. An orange that has gone through the blender does not require any chewing either. The fiber has been ground down into pieces that are functional and small. The sugars and nutrients are absorbed at a slower rate because of the soluble fiber. When you eat an orange, you have to chew the pieces; the stomach has to churn them; and the intestines have to liquefy them so that the fiber pieces are made small enough for absorption of the nutrients to take place.

When it comes to chewing, most nutritionists recommend 20 to 50 chews for each bite. However, a lot of people do not chew more than 10 times, and some fail to chew their food more than three times per bite. This might keep your jaws from having to work, but it passes the buck on to the rest of your digestive system. When you chew your food thoroughly, your digestive tract does not have to work nearly as hard to get the nutrients out. If you chew poorly, complete digestion does not always happen, which means you do not get all of the nutrients out of the food that you are consuming.

In the West, most people eat far too fast because they are eating in the car, eating in a hurry, or eating in front of a television program. If you tried to chew all of your bites 50 times, your jaw will be tired. Many of the conditions and digestive disorders that we have at least in part stem from poor habits when it comes to chewing.

When you blend or juice a fruit or vegetable, you get a supply of nutrients that is both predigested and openly available. The primary difference is that the fiber present in a smoothie slows your body's absorption of the sugars and nutrients. This means that the juice advantage over a smoothie occurs when a person's systems are extremely weak or otherwise not in optimal condition.

If your body is operating normally, smoothies offer quite a few advantages, beginning with fiber. The recommended consumption target for fiber is 25 to 30 grams each day; some nutritionists suggest that this number should be as high as 45. In the United States, though, the average fiber consumption ranges between 12 and 18 grams; in the United Kingdom matters are even worse, as the average range falls between 12 and 16 grams.

Australia is a little bit better, with an average consumption of 20 grams of fiber each day. The Western countries feature high rates of colon cancers, constipation, Type 2 diabetes and high cholesterol; each of these conditions requires a higher level of dietary fiber in order to improve.

Another advantage of the smoothie is that it is filling enough to serve as a meal. The most common meal for a smoothie is breakfast, and since most people are rushing around in the morning, that's a great time to drink one.
If you use a masticating juicer, the process can take as long as half an hour and you still have to clean the machine. This is frustrating for everyone who likes to use a juicer. Centrifugal juicers are faster, but they still take longer than a blender, particularly if you factor in time for cleaning.

Smoothies also produce virtually no waste. You will have some peels from bananas, oranges and other fruits, and you will have some tough green stalks occasionally, but when you juice, you have all of the leftover fiber to deal with. Juices, in contrast, are generally not filling. If you have a special juice as your breakfast, you will be hungry 45 minutes later.

If you drink commercially manufactured juices that come from raw ingredients, you usually have to drink it with a meal. The high sugar content in most juices means that you're taking in calories you don't need. Juices don't have any fiber, so they run right out of the stomach and send sugars into your bloodstream in overdrive. You'll get a jolt of energy, but the crash will be coming later. Consuming a drink with fiber, such as with a smoothie, keeps your blood sugar level on a more even keel and helps you maintain weight control.

If you drink greens in a smoothie, your blood sugar balance stays more stable. You have more fiber in your beverage than you would get just from eating a whole fruit, and the protein present in greens slows down your body's processing of carbohydrates. This means that your blood sugar level stays stable for a longer period of time and you'll feel fewer hunger pangs in between meals.

3: Getting Started

You can use any blender to make a green smoothie (or any other kind of smoothie), but if you are committed to smoothies over the long haul, a durable one is worth the extra green (no pun intended) you will put down to buy one. Blendtec and Vitamix are two brands that earn consistently positive reviews, although they are pricey. A simple food processor will not work for a smoothie, but a multipurpose appliance like the Thermomix will.

In order to incorporate the dietary fiber effectively, you have to run the blender on a green smoothie a little longer than you do with a fruit smoothie. You need a heavy-duty blade to break veggies like celery down and the higher fiber parts of fruit, such as pineapple cores. These blenders should be able to crush ice easily, so that the blended liquid will stay at a low temperature.

If you don't include ice, a smoothie that you blend for a minute will be warm; after two minutes, they are almost hot. This is why some heavy duty blenders are marketed for their ability to generate soup that is steaming hot just from the blade friction. However, warm smoothies are not enjoyable, and the heat can erode the effectiveness of enzymes and nutrients.

Advice for Blending Green Smoothies

- Do you sense a burning smell, or is the base of your blender warm? It's time to give it a rest.

- If you chop your ingredients into smaller pieces before you dump them into the blender, you'll put less wear on the motor and the blade.

- Make sure you put enough liquid in to give the solids room to move. The thicker the smoothie, the more stress on the blade and motor.

- Stay away from frozen ingredients whenever possible, because the motor and blades might not be able to deal with them. If you do use frozen ingredients, cut them into small segments before putting them into the blender.

On the other hand, smoothies that are really cold aren't that good for you either. Traditional Ayurvedic and Chinese medical practices teach that consuming very cold drinks and foods is not a good idea. They consider digestion as being warm, increasing activity in the stomach.

Eating and drinking cold things is said to slow down digestion and take unnecessary energy to heat the food up to the temperature of your body. If you eat something that is frozen, rather than just really cold, this would compound the issue. There is also some research indicating that using very cold ingredients can hinder your body's ability to absorb vitamin B12 and other nutrients.

So what if you only have frozen fruit on hand? If you don't want a super-cold smoothie, use water that is a little warmer. Here are some reminders before you begin your green smoothie diet.

If you are looking to make healthy eating a permanent part of your life, rather than just a phase, then a green smoothie cleanse is a great way to begin. If you can take the toxic burden away from your liver for a week and fill your digestive tract with nutrients, you will feel amazing, and you will want more. Many holistic nutritionists recommend going through this type of cleanse several times each year to give your body a sense of renewal and recharging.

While a green smoothie cleanse is a great idea just about all year long, if you are pregnant, it is not a good idea. The cleanse does have a great deal of nutrients and is nutritionally balanced, but it is also a time of detoxification. Those toxins can enter your bloodstream – as well as your breast milk. So if you are pregnant or nursing, you can incorporate the occasional green smoothie or other recipes in your diet but do not do the cleanse.

One reason why processed foods are so popular is that they are cheap. Boxes of meal helpers and packages of pasta are not as expensive as proteins, fruits and vegetables. So you can expect your grocery bill to jump a bit. However, since you won't be eating out as much either, you can expect this to level off a bit.

But even if your bill goes up a little, it's important to remember that you are making an investment in your health, and you are definitely worth the expense. Here's how I view it: you can pay a little more now on the front end for fresh produce and whole foods that are real, or you can pay on the back end with medical bills when you develop some of the chronic conditions that the Western diet tends to produce.

If you think that type 2 diabetes later on will be cheaper than buying more produce now, you have not been paying attention to the health care debate. After you have bought your staple ingredients, if you want to stick with a regular cleansing regimen, you will find that they last a long time, keeping your monthly expenses lower.

It takes less time to prepare a batch of smoothies and clean the blender than it does to figure out what everyone wants on their pizzas and calling in a delivery order. It takes a LOT less time to make those smoothies than it does to cook a pot full of pasta, let alone put together a full family meal. If you put together a weekly shopping list and have your green smoothie items on hand, then you can get this done.

Everyone's body is different. The basic formula for weight loss is calories in minus calories out – if you burn more calories than you take in, you will lose weight. If you don't, then you will gain weight or stay at the same weight. Your genetics, metabolism, exercise routine, fluid balance and past history all play a part. Weight is also a function of stress for many people, and changing a dietary routine can involve stress for anyone.

However, it's important to remember that this cleanse revolves around giving your body a completely fresh start and you want to find the best version of yourself possible. If you're looking to see a long lasting transformation, it will take way longer than seven days. One thing that you can be sure of is that the differences you feel from having this cleanse will boost your energy level.

Some people wonder whether it's all right to work out during a cleanse and this is something that really varies with the individual. For many people, the smoothie cleans leads to a huge boost in energy. If this pertains to you, then take advantage of it. However, you may find that you are not able to maintain your normal level of intensity, particularly as the week goes by. Just slow down a bit if needed.

This is a question that only your health care provider can answer for you. Many cleanse routines are not recommended for diabetics. However, if you want to give it a try, set up an appointment with your physician to see if this would be acceptable with your condition. Different diabetics have different needs. Even if your doctor doesn't want you doing the full cleanse, incorporating a green smoothie now and then is still a good idea.

4: Dietary Concerns about Green Smoothies

If you're new to vegetarian thinking (and new to green smoothies) you may wonder how you're going to get enough protein during your cleanse. The simple answer as with any other balanced diet is that you will get it from the food that you take in.

Remember, you're starting out on a weeklong cleanse, not a lifetime diet that only consists of green smoothies and similar recipes. It is possible to make a lifelong meal regimen that consists of a couple of green smoothies a day and a high-protein third meal. However, during the cleanse, you're not going to run low on protein.

Also, there is minimal risk of suffering from protein deficiency if your diet consists of a variety of foods that are rich in nutrients. The real task when putting together a lifelong diet is making sure that your meals are rich in nutrients overall; this principle is true if you are vegan, vegetarian, or omnivorous. As long as you have a balanced diet and get all of the nutrients you require, your health will remain sound.

According to the World Health Organization, people only need 10 percent of their calories from protein. The Western diet pushes that up to a third of all calories. Dr. T. Colin Campbell, a professor at Cornell University specializing in nutritional biochemistry, suggests that we really only need 5 or 6 percent to come from protein. However, he recommends the full 10 percent to ensure that we absorb the smaller amount.

What about carbohydrates? In the Western diet, people get almost half, if not more, of their calories from carbs. A lot of the fad diets focus on hitting the protein and depriving the body of carbohydrates, changing the body over to the use of ketones for energy (from fats) rather than carbohydrates. A risk of this sort of change is that a diet that high in protein can lead to such issues as osteoporosis, mood disorders, kidney stones, and even unpleasant body odor. While a high protein diet generally leads to weight loss (usually because of sheer calorie deprivation) and the fact that a set volume of protein is more filling than that same volume of carbohydrates.

If you want to lose weight and maintain an even keel with your blood sugar levels, you need some protein with each meal. Plant sources that are rich in protein are easy to find and include green leaves, alfalfa and lentil sprouts, almonds, sesame seeds, chickpeas and other legumes, and quinoa and other seed grains.

Meat-based protein sources contain all of the necessary amino acids, while plant-based protein sources sometimes lack them. Back in the 1960s, a myth arose that it was not healthy to have a vegetarian meal unless you combined vegetables to find all of the essential amino acids. However, as early as the 1970s, nutritionists found that this combination was not necessary at each meal, or even over the course of each day, as long as you regularly take in a healthy variety of protein.

But what are amino acids? These are the basic building blocks that make up protein. When you eat foods with protein, your digestive tract breaks the proteins down into amino acids and then puts them back together to make new proteins, including the enzymes that your body needs to undertake processes. All in all, there are 22 different amino acids.

Your body needs them all, but it can make 14 of them. The other eight though, you have to consume through your diet. The complete proteins have all of the eight essential acids. However, most sources of concentrated protein have been cooked, a process that eradicates half of the protein available. Even though that source of protein may have been complete at one time, once you prepare it only half of it is available for use.

If you eat raw plant sources of protein, you lose none of the protein, so it is all available. Some plants, like chia, quinoa, amaranth and soy, contain all eight essential amino acids as well. So if you make a green smoothie that is 40 percent green, you've put together a dynamite protein source. Greens are rich in protein; if they weren't, sheep, cattle and apes would not ripple with muscles, and they are vegan.

When you eat some spinach, 30 percent of your calories come from protein. This is a higher ratio than the protein-based calories in cheese (26 percent) and whole milk (23 percent). While the ratio in beef is 50 percent, remember that cooking eradicates half of protein, so if you eat 4 ounces of cooked beef, that's the same available protein as what you would get from 3.2 ounces of raw spinach.

The Skinny on Carbs

If you pick up just about any diet book in the West, you might easily conclude that if we could just eliminate carbohydrates from the planet, all of our weight problems would go away. It is true that the world is increasing in its overall obesity, but it is simplistic to blame the carbohydrate for all of the dietary problems on the planet.

Just like not all proteins are the same, not all carbs are the same either. When you read the fine print on some of those low carb diets out there, they generally refer to sugar and carbs with starch. Many of those diets allow you to keep eating fruit (a source of the sugar fructose), and some of them allow you to keep eating grains.

But just what are carbohydrates in the first place? From a technical standpoint, they are just saccharides. All this term means is that oxygen, hydrogen and carbon appear in their molecular makeup. Within the carbohydrate family is a wide variety of structures though varying from the simple to the complex.

The sweeter monosaccharides, such as fructose and glucose are simple as are the disaccharides (two molecules linked) like sucrose, which is table sugar and consists of fructose and glucose combined. Then you get the oligosaccharides, which do not taste sweet and consist of more complex sugar molecule chains. These are foods like beans. You also get the polysaccharides which are lengthy strings of the smaller forms; glycogen, starch and cellulose are three types of these. If you want to get energy out of your carbs though, your body must break them down into one of the monosaccharide forms. Until then, your body will not be able to use these for energy.

The carbohydrate that you find in the bloodstream is glucose which gives you immediate energy in the tissues and cells. The liver metabolizes fructose and stores it in the form glycogen releasing it as needed into your bloodstream as glucose. If you take in too much fructose, the body metabolizes it as fat. One possible destination is storage in the liver, although that can lead to unhealthy condition known as fatty liver.

Among natural sweeteners, sweet foods such as cane sugar or sucrose provide energy both up front in a short burst as well as through a slower release. Complex carbs, such as the starches you find in root vegetables and grains that have undergone processing have many glucose molecules linked together. They require more time to break down than sweets, but they also provide a relatively high level of fuel based in glucose.

The most complex carbs, such as fiber do not break down into absorbable units and simply leave the body through the bowel, carrying other things along with them in a very healthy process. The starches that appear in nature, like in root vegetables also have fiber in them. When you eat those as a whole food, they will slow the process down whereby the body absorbs glucose right in the bloodstream.

When it comes to choosing carbohydrates, the primary problems come from processing and refining. The natural design for carbohydrates includes forms that operate for the benefit of your body. There are some fruits that are very sweet, like watermelon, but even the sweetest fruits have a healthy balance of simple sugars.

Vegetables and grains provide a healthy balance of the fiber and starch. When you open a box of breakfast cereal that has been processed, the essential fibers, fats and vitamins have been leached out and all that remains is a starchy glob of carbohydrate sending you a quick dose of glucose.

One reason why the sugary soft drinks are so unhealthy is that the high fructose corn syrup gives the liver an overload of fructose. However, when you eat whole fruits along with a healthy balance of grains and vegetables, you get the nutritional balance that the body is supposed to have (assuming that you are not gluten or fructose intolerant).

A lot of people just want to eliminate carbs from their dietary plans, or at least reduce them. If you look at this from a strict standpoint, getting rid of all carbs would mean a diet without any sugar, grains, fruits, vegetables or legumes. You would just get protein and fat from meat, nuts, eggs and dairy.

This sort of diet would cause significant problems as nutritional deficiencies would accumulate. If you're really interested in monitoring your carb intake, look at the glycemic index (GI) or glycemic load (GL) for a particular food. Managing your diet on a case-by-case basis is much more helpful to the body than simply trying to ban all carbs from the body.

So what is actually important with regard to your carbs? The type of carb you're taking in is just as important as your caloric count. This means that while you will want to eliminate as many donuts from your diet, carbs from sources like fruits and vegetables are a different matter.

5: Getting the Most out of Each Smoothie

One question that many people have about putting together a green smoothie has to do with the combination of food. Some people don't know whether it is all right to combine vegetables and fruits in a smoothie. I personally believe that there is a difference between greens and other vegetables – and that difference is starch content. Just like there is a difference between chicken and eggs, even though they both come from the same source, I believe that there is a considerable differentiation between what vegetables are and what greens are.

To me, the "greens" are the flat plant leaves that are connected to the stem. These are not the starchy parts of the plants. Also, "greens" are not fruits that have yet to turn their natural color because of a lack of ripeness. While a lot of people know better than to buy green bananas, there are some people who buy green apples, limes, melons and green grapes in the thought that those are "greens."

If you eat fruit that isn't ripe yet, you can get irritation in your intestines because of some of the substances those fruits contain. Also, those fruits generally have more starch and less sugar, making digestion tougher.

Adding actual greens to other foods, though, provides quite a few benefits. Greens have a great deal of fiber as well as the other nutritional advantages. The fiber slows down the process of absorbing sugar, which is why green smoothies are all right for people to drink, even when they are highly sensitive to sugar. This is why it is all right for diabetics to incorporate the smoothies into their diets, even though cleanses can be more difficult.

So how can you get the most out of each smoothie that you make? Here are some tips that have worked well.

- Make your green smoothies at the beginning of the day. You can make a quart or two – enough for your entire day of cleansing. Store what you don't drink right away in the refrigerator. However, freezing smoothies generally does not work.

- Sip slowly as you enjoy your smoothie. Allow your saliva to get into the smoothie as well while you swallow so that your absorption will go more smoothly. If you're not quite finished with it when it's time to head to work, you can pour it into a travel cup and take it with you.

- If nuts, oils, seeds or powder supplements tend to irritate you, it is all right to stick to fruit, greens and water. Many people find the irritation takes place in the form of discomfort and unwanted gas.

- Don't incorporate the smoothie into a larger meal, even after you're done with the cleanse. Instead, make the smoothie a standalone meal. This will give you the most benefit from your green smoothie nutritionally. Wait about 45 minutes after you have finished your smoothie before you eat anything else.

- Starchy vegetables like green beans, corn, peas, okra, squash, pumpkin, eggplant, cabbage, cauliflower, zucchini, broccoli stems, beets and carrots are all likely to contribute gas to your digestive tract if you include them in your smoothies. This is just a friendly warning.

- Keep experimenting with new combinations in your green smoothies.
  This keeps an element of fun in the process, and it will keep your interest alive. If you get bored with it – or if your smoothies aren't tasty – you will get away from the habit once the cleansing is over.

- Blending time is really going to vary with your ingredients. Usually, it will not take longer than 30 seconds to do the job. However, if you have celery, pomegranate seeds, or mango slices that include the peel, it might take as long as a minute. If you know you have tougher items in the blender, spend the first half minute at a low speed, and then turn the speed up and blend until the texture is consistent and creamy.

- If your blender is a high-speed model, leave the peel on your pears, kiwis, apples and mangoes; the additional fiber will help you out. With pears and apples, you can leave the seeds in – again, you'll get the benefit of fiber and other nutrients. However, if you only have a low speed blender, seeds and peels are likely to wreck the machine. With a pineapple's peel, though, always remove it. Also, if you are using fruit that was not grown according to organic principles, you will want to peel that as well.

- Choose fruits that are rich in pectin and soluble fiber. That way, the texture will be creamy, and your fiber and liquid will stay together. The best choices are blueberries, strawberries, peaches, pears, bananas and mangoes.

- If you get froth in a smoothie, the likely cause is apple that has not yet blended thoroughly. If you don't like froth in your smoothie, think about incorporating an avocado pit. These have a lot of soluble fiber, so if you put half a pit in for each 32 ounces of smoothie you want, you'll get less froth; just make sure you are using a high speed blender, and toss the pit in after you have started the blender with your other ingredients so that you don't wreck the blade.

- Take the stalks off chard, collards and kale before you start blending. They tend to add a peppery flavor that can be unpleasant. For cilantro, parsley, dandelions and spinach, though, you can leave the stalks on. You'll get more fiber without the impact on the flavor.

- There are some recipes that ask for coconut meat and water. Check below for some instructions on the best way to prepare all of that.

Handling Coconut

When you are selecting your coconuts, pick out the young ones. They have almost a liter of water, and they are the healthiest ones for eating. As coconuts mature, the jelly inside them begins to harden into flesh, costing you some of the nutritional benefits. Shake a coconut to see if it is good; choose ones that are heavy. If you can hear water splashing around, you'll know that some of the water has started to harden, because there will be air inside to allow the water to move.

When you're ready to open a coconut, start by putting it on one side, with the top (the pointed end) facing away from you. Use a large knife with a serrated blade to start shaving the husk away from the coconut's point, revealing the shell.

Turn the coconut as necessary, and keep cutting the husk off, moving completely around the point. Beneath the white husk you will see a shell that is light brown. When you buy a coconut in a store, this husk has already been taken off. If you shave the husk off in a full circle, you will have an easier time opening the coconut.

Put your knife just on the inside of the circle you've made. Use the knife to stab the shell and make a crack; this should take the shape of a sphere, because coconut shells feature a grain that is round. Cut an inch or so into the coconut shell, and then slice down a couple more inches through the shell.

Now set the coconut with the pointed side facing up; if you don't, the water will run out of the coconut. Give the knife a slight twist, and you will see a circular opening forming at the top. When you have separated the top halfway from the remainder of the shell, pick up the top completely with your hands.

If you use the coconut water but want to set aside the meat for later, put the top of the coconut back on top and set it in the fridge for no longer than four days. When you're ready to take the meat out, you can just scoop it right out with a spoon. The softer and thinner the meat is, the younger the coconut. If you notice that the coconut meat has turned pinkish, the fermentation process has begun. This usually does not mean that the coconut has spoiled, but you will notice a slightly different flavor. If you are worried about whether the coconut has started to spoil, just throw it away.

Also, don't be afraid to add herbs to your smoothies. A lot of greens either have no flavor at all or a faint bitterness that the fruit has to balance. Herbs not only add some vibrant flavor to your green smoothie, but they also add in a number of benefits, both medicinally and nutritionally.

There are literally hundreds of different herb species with thousands of varieties and subspecies available all around the world in gardens, as well as what you can find growing in the wild. However, four are particularly commonplace in green smoothies: mint, parsley, cilantro and basil. They all help with digestion; they all fight inflammation and bacteria; they all help you fend off cancer. Vitamins A, C, K are in all four of them, as are iron, calcium, manganese and folic acid. Vitamin C is an antioxidant that helps support the immune system as well as healing in the soft tissues. Vitamin K is crucial for healthy bones and consistent blood clotting. Vitamin A is an antioxidant that helps keep your eyes healthy. Folic acid is actually in the "B" family of vitamins, and it has a number of benefits. It helps babies develop neurologically; it helps our cells reproduce DNA accurately; and it keeps our moods stable. Iron appears in hemoglobin within the red blood cells. Calcium is crucial to maintain strong bone structure and for keeping muscle contractions normal. Manganese facilitates reactions among enzymes within the body.

Mint

The name "mint" goes back to Greek mythology. The God of the underworld, Hades, fell in love with Minthe, a beautiful nymph. Hades' wife, Persephone, became jealous of Minthe and cast a spell on her, transforming her into a plant that she could trample on. Hades could not reverse the effects of the spell but did give Minthe a scent that would become stronger the more people stepped on it. This is the classic menthol odor of peppermint.

Common varieties of mint include chocolate mint, pineapple mint, apple mint, peppermint and spearmint. Its aroma helps with concentration and memory. Menthol works as a mild pain reliever for the skin and is frequently included in topical lotions for easing muscular pain. Mint also has cleansing and antibacterial properties, which is why you often find it in products designed for oral hygiene.

Mint also has several organic compounds such as rosmarinic acid, which fights inflammation in your airways; and perillyl alcohol, which helps fight tumors. Mint has vitamin E, vitamin B2, magnesium and potassium. It blends will with cilantro, basil, citrus, kiwi, ginger, cucumber, tomato, parsley, melon, lemon and lime.

Parsley

Parsley is actually related to carrots and celery. In ancient Greeks, the winners of athletic contests were adorned with parsley. It has a great deal of chlorophyll, a green pigment that chelates or detoxifies heavy metals while also masking the odors of other foods. If you chew some parsley after you eat a meal made with something like garlic, you will have fresher breath. Parsley also contains a great deal of antioxidant flavonoids and vitamins. Luteolin is one of these flavonoids; it fights cancer and gets rid of other toxins in the blood. Myristicin is an oil inside parsley that boosts the work of glutathione, one of the liver's most important antioxidants.

Parsley also has zeathanthin, a carotene pigment that is vital for healthy vision. Because of its high concentrations of iron and vitamin C, parsley is beneficial for vegetarians. The iron from plants is tougher for the body to process than iron from animal foods, but vitamin C makes iron uptake more efficient.

Cilantro

If you live in the United Kingdom, you probably know cilantro (the name in the Americas) as coriander. Either way, the leaves have been a popular supplement for thousands of years, dating all the way back to the regimens of the Sanskrit and Egyptian physicians.

Cilantro has many of the usual herbal benefits, such as power against inflammation, anxiety, bacteria and cancer, and it also helps significantly with digestion. However, it has additional benefits for diabetics, as it regulates the activity of insulin in the body. It also helps the body process fat, leading to less accumulation of the unhealthy forms of cholesterol.

Cilantro does have a strong flavor in comparison to other herbs, and most people will either hate or love cilantro. If the flavor is a bit much for you, you can blend it with parsley or mint to tame the taste a bit. The high levels of chlorophyll mean that it will chelate toxins and heavy metals right out of your body. Cilantro is rich in quercetin, a flavonoid that fights inflammation, allergies and viruses.

In green smoothies, the flavor of cilantro blends well with pineapple, parsley, mint, lime, lemon, kiwi, ginger, cucumber, coconut, beet, basil and avocado.

Basil

The name "basil" comes from the Greek term for "royal," and this herb is the Italian symbol for love. It is genetically related to mint and works like peppermint and spearmint medicinally.

Basil helps control spasms in the small intestine by relaxing the smooth musculature within those walls. It dilates smaller blood vessels helping to boost circulation. It is also viewed as a helpful agent to fight worms. It has a warming effect on smoothies and other foods and can taste like cloves. In a green smoothie, basil blends will with tomato, mint, lime, lemon, ginger, fig, coconut milk and cilantro.

6: Smoothie Recipes for a Beginner

For all of these, blend for 30 seconds and check for a creamy, consistent texture. If the smoothies have celery, pomegranate seeds, or peel, start at a low speed for 20 to 30 seconds and then turn it up higher for the last 20 or 30 seconds.

Morning Balance

1 cup kale
1 mango
1 cup water

Yield: 1 quart

Morning Energy Jolt

½ bunch dandelion greens
½ inch fresh ginger root
2 celery stalks
2 peaches
½ pineapple (remove the peel first!)

Yield: 2 quarts

Parsley Cantaloupe Delight

3 cups cantaloupe, cubed
1 bunch parsley, fresh

Yield: 1 quart

Passionate Parsley Smoothie

1 bunch parsley, fresh
1 Fuji apple (only peel and core if you have a low speed blender)
1 ripe banana
1 cucumber, peeled
1-2 cups water (the more water, the thinner the texture)

Yield: 2 quarts

Dandelion Surprise

2 mangoes
2 cups apple juice
1 bunch dandelion greens
2 pears
1 cup water

Yield: 2 quarts

Spring Dandelion

2 cups apple juice
3 cups dandelion greens, freshly picked
1 fresh mango
1 cup water
1 ripe peach

Yield: 2 quarts

Absolutely Peachy

1 head butter lettuce

3 peaches
2 cups water
½ pint raspberries

Yield: 2 quarts

Watermelon Delight

1 banana
4 cups fresh watermelon chunks (no rind!)
Juice from ½ lemon
5 leaves romaine lettuce

Yield: 2 quarts

Poppin' Papaya Smoothie

1 banana
1 fresh papaya, without the seeds
2 cups spinach
1 cup water

Yield: 1 quart

Melon Medallions Smoothie

9 leaves romaine lettuce
3 cups cantaloupe, cubed

Yield: 1 quart

Black Currant Bliss

1 ripe mango
1 pint black currants

1 head butter lettuce
2 cups orange juice

Yield: 2 quarts

The Mixin' Mango

2 cups water
2 mangos
1 cup spinach

Yield: 1 quart

Soulful Strawberry Smoothie

1 cup strawberries
1 cup romaine lettuce
1 banana
1 cup water

Yield: 1 quart

Tropical Tuesday Smoothie

2 cups water
1 cup mixed baby leaves
1 cup pineapple (no peel!)
1 mango

Yield: 1 quart

Twilight Delight

2 cups water
1 cup spinach

1 banana
1 cup pineapple (no peel!)

Yield: 1 quart

Particularly Pear Smoothie

2 cups water
1 cup spinach
1 banana
2 pears

Yield: 1 quart

The Frugal Gourmet (with apologies)

1 cup water
½ cucumber
1 banana
2 apples

Yield: 1 quart

Sweet Surprise

1 cup spinach
1 mango
1 cup strawberries
2 cups water
Yield: 1 quart

Peachy Pie

2 celery stalks

1 banana
3 peaches
1 cup water
Yield: 1 quart

Blissful Blueberry Smoothie

1 cup spinach
1 banana
1 cup blueberries
2 cups water

Yield: 1 quart

Rippling Raspberry Smoothie

2 cups water
1 cup bok choy OR pak choi
1 banana
1 cup raspberries

Yield: 1 quart

The Best Berry Ever

1 cup spinach
1 mango
1 cup mixed berries
2 cups water

Yield: 1 quart

Cool Citrus Surprise

1 cup spinach
1 orange
1 cup pineapple
1 cup water

Yield: 1 quart

Apricot Amazement

1 cup romaine lettuce
1 banana
1 cup apricots
2 cups water

Yield: 1 quart

Coconut Craze

1 cup spinach
½ cup coconut
1 pineapple
1 cup water

Yield: 1 quart

7: The Greatness of Fruit Flavors

Yes, these are all "green" smoothies, but each one of these has fruit greatness that you will taste. They won't necessarily look fruity, but you will love the flavors.

Acai

The acai berry is indigenous to South and Central America, and it grows on the acai palm tree. People who love these berries say they taste like a blending of chocolate and red wine.

When you put it into a green smoothie, it works well as an accent taste for other tropical flavors, such as papaya and banana (these are some of the base fruits that make smoothies creamy). Acai also tastes pleasant with pear and apple.

Acai berries have a great deal of antioxidants, and their phytonutrients help to fight diseases. There are some marketers who hype acai as the cure for cancer, the end of diabetes and the magic fruit for weight loss; those claims still have yet to be proven. Also, you will find just as many antioxidants in Concord grapes and black cherries, so this is not a magic food from the tropics. However, the acai berry is definitely something to work into your green smoothie arsenal. You can't buy them fresh in Europe or North America, so look for frozen acai berry purees, which you will find on websites like Amafruits.com or in some health food stores or specialty grocers.

Why purees? You can also find acai as a powder or juice, but those products have gone through more processing and there is a higher risk of oxidization. Also, whole food puree is available more economically than the powders, extracts or juices, which are packaged (and priced) as supplements.

If you try to use acai juice as the liquid for your smoothie, you'll find the flavor is a bit strong. This is why the puree works well. Now, here are some smoothie recipes with the acai berry.

Acai Super Antioxidant Blast with Pomegranate

100 grams of acai berry puree, frozen
½ cup fresh pomegranate arils
½ cup blueberries
1 banana, peeled
8 ounces unsweetened almond milk

Add the liquids first, and then the fruit.

Yield: 16 ounces

Acai/Blueberry/Strawberry Blended Smoothie

½ cup blueberries
10 strawberries

100 grams acai berry puree, frozen OR 1 ounce
acai berry juice
3 cups baby kale
1 banana, peeled
8 ounces almond milk, unsweetened
1 tablespoon cacao powder

Add the liquids first, and then the fruit.

Yield: 16 ounces

Apple

It seems like the claim "an apple a day keeps the
doctor away" is as old as time itself. However,
researchers keep finding more and more reasons to
make apples a staple in your diet. Some studies
show that pregnant woman should eat apples, as it
can lower their risk of having children who later
come down with asthma. Also, there are some
studies that show that apple juice can guard against
wheezing in children.
The best type of apple to buy is one that is in
season. If you live in North America, they are best
between September and December, although
different varieties are available at different times of
the year.

Apples rank #2 for residue of pesticides, according
to a study by the Environmental Working Group.
So you definitely want to buy organic apples when

possible, and if not, you want to wash those apples thoroughly before you put them into your blender (or your mouth).

Apple skin is chock full of nutrients and fiber and definitely belongs in your green smoothie. (This is why cleaning it is so important!)

Apple Lemon Smoothie

2 apples
2 cups fresh baby spinach (substitute another leafy green if desired)
1 whole carrot
½ lemon (juiced)
½ cup water

Yield: 16 ounces

Apple Grape Smoothie

1 apple
1 cup red grapes
1 whole carrot
½ cup water
2 cups fresh baby spinach (substitute another leafy green if desired)
Yield: 16 ounces

Apple Banana Pear Smoothie

1 apple
1 pear

1 banana
1 stalk of celery
½ cup water
2 cups fresh baby spinach (substitute another leafy green if desired)

Yield: 16 ounces

Apple Blueberry Smoothie

1 apple
2 cups fresh baby spinach (substitute another leafy green if desired)
1 cup blueberries
¼ avocado
½ cup water
Yield: 16 ounces

Green Apple

2 apples
2 cups fresh baby spinach (substitute another leafy green if desired)
1 celery stalk (if desired)
½ cup water

Yield: 16 ounces

Apricot

The apricot is a fruit that is both tart and sweet. They look a lot like peaches, but they are not as big, and they have a smoother skin. It is hard for them to grow in North America because of our uneven climate, but in their indigenous regions of China and Armenia, they grow quite well.

If you have a green smoothie in the summer and incorporate strawberries, watermelons, nectarines, or peaches, apricots can complement the tastes quite nicely. Apricots also blend well with such tropical fruits as the coconut.

As you might expect, apricots are teeming with vitamin C. However, they also have the amino acid tryptophan, so they can help complete the protein in a dietary day. The carotenoids in apricots make them a preventer of cardiac disease and help you reduce your cholesterol levels. Some studies have shown that apricots can help you with vision and keep you from experiencing constipation. The lycopene in an apricot may help keep you from developing prostate cancer as well.

Choose an apricot that is rich in its orange hue and just a bit soft. If they are yellow or pale, stay away from them, because they are not ripe yet. They will appear in supermarkets between May and August.

So take a look at some of these recipes:

Apricot Strawberry Smoothie

2-4 apricots
1 apple

1 whole carrot
½ cup strawberries
2 cups fresh baby spinach (substitute another leafy green if desired)
½ cup water

Yield: 16 ounces

Apricot Ginger Smoothie

2-4 apricots
1 tablespoon ginger, to taste
2 cups fresh baby spinach (substitute another leafy green if desired)
1 small celery stalk
1 apple

Yield: 16 ounces

Apricot Peach Smoothie

2 apricots
2 cups fresh baby spinach (substitute another leafy green if desired)
1 whole carrot
1 peach
½ cup water

Yield: 16 ounces

Apricot Banana Smoothie

2-4 apricots

2 cups fresh baby spinach (substitute another leafy green if desired)
1 whole banana
½ cup water

Yield: 16 ounces

Blackberry

Blackberries are one of the more versatile fruits, making appearances on plates raw but also showing up in wines, jams, candies and desserts. In the United States, Oregon is the leading center of blackberry production, and no country grows more blackberries than the U.S.

When it comes to flavor, the blackberry is sweeter than tart, and it draws comparisons to raspberries. Blackberries are smoother than raspberries (red or black varieties), and they do not feature any hair. Also, a blackberry holds onto its stem after you pick it, while a raspberry does not.

There are only few fruits that have more antioxidants than blackberries. Blackberries have a great deal of vitamin C, copper, manganese and fiber. They also contain high amounts of folate, vitamins A, B5, C, E and K, as well as zinc. The phytochemical cyandin-3-glucoside appears in blackberries and may help in the fight against cancer.

Now, take a look at these recipes that incorporate blackberries:

Black and Blue Smoothie

1 cup blackberries
2-4 cups fresh baby spinach (substitute another leafy green if desired)
2-4 ounces filtered water
1 banana, peeled
1 cup watermelon (no rind!)

Yield: 16 ounces

Blackberry Orange Smoothie

1 cup blackberries
1 small orange, peeled and seeded
2 cups fresh baby spinach (substitute another leafy green if desired)
1 banana, peeled
8 ounces filtered water

Yield: 16 ounces

Blackberry Mango Smoothie

1 cup blackberries
1 vine tomato
2 cups fresh baby spinach (substitute another leafy green if desired)
1 large mango, pitted and peeled
 8 ounces filtered water

Yield: 16 ounces

Blackberry Melon Surprise

1 cup blackberries
1 banana, peeled
1 cup watermelon
2-4 fresh baby spinach (substitute another leafy green if desired)
2-4 ounces filtered water

Yield: 16 ounces

Checkerboard Smoothie

½ cup raspberries
½ cup blackberries
2 cups fresh baby spinach (substitute another leafy green if desired)
2 bananas, peeled
1 celery stalk (if desired)
8 ounces filtered water

Yield: 16 ounces

Blackberry Veggie Apple Smoothie

1 cup blackberries
2 cups fresh baby spinach (substitute another leafy green if desired)
2 small apples, cored
1 small carrot
1 celery stalk (if desired)

8 ounces filtered water

Yield: 16 ounces

Blueberry

This is one of the most popular summer fruits, cultivated between May and August in the United States. However, they are available in the frozen food aisle all year long in most grocery stores.

Blueberries have long been a staple in North America. Long before the Europeans showed up to colonize the Americas, Native Americans prized them. Not only were they a valued food, but they also were used in medicines and as clothing dyes. The United States produces more than 90 percent of the blueberries in the world today.

The flavoring in blueberries is sweet and consistent, and you can add them to most smoothies to enhance the taste. They are high in the antioxidants that prevent some cancers and fight inflammation. They are also high in vitamins B6, C and K, as well as dietary fiber and manganese. Their glycemic load is relatively low among fruits, which means you can eat them without having to go through a spike in blood sugar.

Some studies indicate that eating blueberries (as well as cranberries) can ameliorate the cognitive erosion that takes place with Alzheimer's disease as well as other conditions that are generally related to age. They also help prevent infections in the urinary tract.

When you are shopping for blueberries, they may come pre-packaged in plastic cartons. Look through the sides of the carton to check for berries that are leaking or have a whitish mold growing on them. If you buy frozen blueberries, look for the word "wild" on the label. If you can find those, you will get more phytonutrients in your blueberries.

Take a look at some of these recipes that are centered on the deliciousness of the blueberry.

Blueberry Peach Smoothie

1 cup blueberries
¼ avocado
1 celery stalk (if desired)
1 peach
2 cups fresh baby spinach (substitute another leafy green if desired)
½ cup water

Yield: 16 ounces

Blueberry Apple Smoothie

1 cup blueberries
2 cups fresh baby spinach (substitute another leafy green if desired)

1 apple
¼ avocado
½ cup water

Yield: 16 ounces

Blueberry Banana Smoothie

1 cup blueberries
2 cups fresh baby spinach (substitute another leafy green if desired)
1 celery stalk (if desired)
1-2 whole bananas, peeled
½ cup water (1 cup if you use 2 bananas)

Yield: 16-24 ounces

Blueberry Mango Smoothie

1 cup blueberries
2 cups fresh baby spinach (substitute another leafy green if desired)
1 whole carrot
1 mango
½ cup water

Yield: 16 ounces

8: More Smoothies with Fruit

Admit it – you were thinking that green smoothies were likely to taste like broccoli. Nothing is further from the truth! Check out even more great green smoothie recipes that center around fruit.

Cactus Pear

This is the fruit that the nopal, or the prickly pear cactus, bears. This is also called the cactus fig and even the tuna (if you are in Latin America). In Mexico, this is a very popular fruit. You can find it in most grocery stores in North America between June and September, as this is a fruit that goes through a summer harvest. The flavor of the cactus pear is sweet; it will remind you of a combination of the kiwi and the watermelon.

Nutritionally, cactus pears have quite a few benefits. They have a lot of fiber, vitamin C and magnesium, as well as a lot of carotenoids and antioxidants. Within Mexican traditions of folk medicine, the juice and pulp of the cactus pear have been used for treating a variety of conditions, such as inflammation and injuries, as well as urinary tract and digestive issues.

Researchers have looked at several different compounds within the prickly pear cactus species for possible use in the treatment of obesity, high cholesterol, colitis, hangover and viral infections. The *Opuntia streptacantha* species has proven to lower blood sugar by as much as 46 percent when you broil and eat the stems (but not the fruity part). However, raw stems of that species do not have the same effect, nor do other prickly pear species.

Warning:

If you have diabetes, you need to talk to your doctor before trying cactus pear. While the varieties that lower blood sugar are rare, as established above, you do not want to end up going into hypoglycemia after your smoothie.

You can use both the fruit and the leaves of the cactus pear in your smoothies. The flavor of the fruit works well with other tropical fruits, and the green leaves (nopals) can replace other leafy greens.

However, watch out for the seeds and the spines. Cactus pear seeds will not pulverize inside a blender, not even the most powerful ones. Instead, your smoothie will contain jagged seed pieces that might lodge in your throat or cause irritation in your intestines. Get the seeds out before you start blending.

One fairly easy way to get these seeds out is to slice the fruit in half and scoop the seeds out to a strainer. Mash the pulp with a spoon into the strainer, sending the juice through and making the fruit easier to split apart from the seeds. Put a metal bowl beneath the strainer, as the juice will leave a stain on plastic. If you peel the fruit, you will ensure that there are no more spines remaining.

When you are shopping, choose cactus pear that are a rich crimson hue and that are slightly soft when you touch them. Be careful for spines that the grocer may not have taken out!

Cactus Pear Pineapple Smoothie

2 cactus pear fruit, seeds and skin removed
2 cups spinach
Juice from half a lime
½ cup pineapple
4 to 6 ounces filtered water

Yield: 16 ounces

Cactus Pear Pomegranate Green smoothie

1 cactus pear fruit, seeds and skin removed
1 small banana
½ cup pomegranate arils
2 cups spinach
4 to 6 ounces freshly squeezed orange juice
Yield: 16 ounces

Cactus Pear Mango Green Smoothie

2 cactus pear fruit, seeds and skin removed
8 ounces coconut water
¼ cup fresh parsley leaves
½ mango, pitted and peeled

Yield: 16 ounces

Orange

Around the globe, oranges are a popular citrus choice. Oranges are the most highly cultivated tree based fruit on the planet, and there are many different varieties, each with its own size and/or flavor. You'll find them year round, but they are really "in season" from October through February in the United States. While Florida has become known for its orange groves, they were not grown in North America until the 1500s. Their origins are in China and Southeast Asia.

You probably know about the vitamin C that you will find in oranges. However, they also are chock full of dietary fiber, calcium, folate, potassium and vitamins A and B1. Studies have shown that eating oranges lowers your blood pressure, reduces your cholesterol levels, and fights inflammation. The fiber and vitamin C are both connected with a lower risk of developing colon cancer. Diets that contain a lot of oranges may also reduce your risk of oral, stomach and esophageal cancers.

When you are shopping for oranges, look for the ones that are brightly colored and are just barely firm. Don't buy oranges that have shriveled, have developed dents or feel too soft to the touch.

When you are preparing the orange for the blender, leave as much of the white parts (the pith) as you can, because this is where an orange's calcium is stored. The peel is also high in nutrients; however, instead of dumping peel into the blender, just grate about a tablespoon off the orange before you peel it. Then add that tablespoon to your smoothie.

Try these recipes to get oranges into your green smoothie routine.

Orange Papaya Smoothie

1 orange
2 cups fresh baby spinach (or other leafy green)
1 papaya
½ cup water

Yield: 16 ounces

Orange Strawberry Banana Smoothie

1 orange
1 banana, peeled
1 cup whole strawberries
½ cup water
2 cups fresh baby spinach (or other leafy green)

Orange Grape Papaya Smoothie

1 orange
1 cup red grapes
1 cup papaya
2 cups fresh baby spinach (or other leafy green)
2 celery stalks
½ cup water

Yield: 16 ounces

Orange Berry Banana Smoothie

1 orange
1 cup raspberries, strawberries or blueberries
¼ avocado
1 banana
2 cups fresh baby spinach (or other leafy green)
½ cup water

Yield: 16 ounces

Orange Red Grape Smoothie

1 orange
1 cup red grapes
1 apple
2 cups fresh baby spinach (or other leafy green)
2 celery stalks
½ cup water
2 celery stalks
½ cup water

Yield: 16 ounces

Pumpkin

Autumn is the season of pumpkins: you see them on porches, both carved and uncarved. You see them incorporated into holiday pies. However, a lot of people don't consider pumpkins when they are thinking about green smoothie ingredients. However, they are quite nutritious, and you can either use raw or cooked pumpkin in your recipe.

Just one cup of mashed pumpkin has more than 400 percent of your recommended allowance of vitamin A. It also has all of the B vitamins, except for B12, and it is also rich in vitamins C and E. Iron, copper, phosphorus, potassium and manganese are also plentiful in pumpkin.

Pumpkin blends well with a number of other flavors and makes an outstanding smoothie base. Some of the best flavor blends include pears, apples, carrot, coconut and yam. Spices like allspice, vanilla, ginger, nutmeg, clove, cinnamon and that eponymous "pumpkin pie spice" all work well, as does raw cacao.

Canned pumpkin is the easiest to use in a smoothie, but make sure that you choose an organic label that does not have any added sugar. Look for "unsweetened organic pumpkin pie mix" or "pure pumpkin puree" on the can.

You can also cut pumpkin up and cook it, letting it chill before you put it in a smoothie. The best method for cooking is steaming. Just take out the seeds and the inner parts, take off the peel, and cut the rest into small sections. Put it in a colander basket or a steamer with a lid on top of boiling water for 45 to 50 minutes, until the meat is tender. You can boil it, but you'll end up losing nutrients into the water. Steamed pumpkin will have the most flavor and nutrients. Don't use more than a cup, though, or the pumpkin will dominate the smoothie.

Check out these green smoothie recipes that incorporate pumpkin.

Pumpkin Carrot and Pear Green Smoothie

1 cup pumpkin
1 whole carrot
1 ripe pear, cored
2 cups fresh baby spinach (or other leafy green)

Yield: 16 ounces

Pumpkin Apple Green Smoothie with Cinnamon

1 cup pumpkin

1 banana, peeled
1 apple, cored
Cinnamon to taste
2 cups fresh baby spinach (or other leafy green)
8 ounces filtered water Yield: 16 ounces

9: Focus on Vegetables

So far, the focus has been on emphasizing fruit in these green smoothies. However, the greens that you choose are also important. This chapter focuses on the nutritional benefits that different greens will bring.

Bok Choy

Bok choy is also known as Chinese cabbage or pak choi, and it is genetically related to kale, broccoli and cabbage. The leaves are flat and dark green, while the stalk is wide, long and white. The leaves are not as soft as spinach or kale, but you will get antioxidants, minerals and vitamins in plenty in your green smoothie.

If you put five leaves of bok choy into your smoothie, you only add nine calories, but you get all of the vitamin A you need for the day. You get a third of the vitamin C and more than a quarter of the vitamin K. You also get 70 mg of calcium.

Bok choy also has glucosinolates, which contain protective properties that may help the body fight cancer cells and cut down on oxidative stress.

It is worth pointing out, though, that if you have a thyroid condition you may not be able to process the glucosinolates appropriately, which can lead to a toxic condition. However, you have to eat a lot of bok choy on a regular basis for this to become a problem. If you include this as a part of your rotation of greens, you will be fine.

The flavor of bok choy leaves is on the bitter side, like a stronger version of spinach. This can be pleasing when you eat it raw, but in a smoothie, it is easy to mask the taste with the fruits that you choose. It is not as bitter as kale and not nearly as bitter as dandelion. If you toss an entire head into a smoothie, you will get the nutritional benefits.

When you are shopping for bok choy, look for leaves that are dark green and stalks that are white and bright, although in baby bok choy the stalks can also be greenish. If the stalks are yellowing at all, stay away from them.

If you have to store bok choy before you use it, put a paper towel or dry cloth in your storage bin. This will absorb the moisture so that your bok choy takes longer to decompose.

Dandelion Greens

Many green smoothie aficionados rate dandelion greens as their top green to throw into a smoothie. They have more iron and calcium than the majority of cultivated greens, and there are several health benefits that make them a nutritional wonder.

- Dandelion greens are loaded with vitamin C, which helps the body absorb iron, and vitamin A, in the form of beta carotene.

- Dandelion greens have more iron than any leafy green except fresh parsley. Just one cup of dandelion greens has 1.7 mg of iron.

- Looking for calcium? Just one cup of dandelion greens has 103 mg of calcium – a tenth of what you need all day. This is more than kale. If you add a couple of cups to a smoothie with papaya, fig, orange or another calcium-rich fruit, your smoothie will have more calcium in it than a glass of milk.

- Dandelion greens are one-seventh protein, and they contain all of the eight essential amino acids. This means that incorporating it in your smoothie knocks out your amino acid needs for the entire day.

- One cup of dandelion greens has 25 calories. This is a little higher than other greens, which makes it a good choice for your morning smoothie, when you want a few more calories.

During the spring and summer, it's likely that you will find plenty of dandelion greens in your yard. However, you can also buy them year-round in farmer's markets and health food stores. If you are shopping, look for leaves that are dark and green without any blemishes. If you are looking in the wild, picking young greens that have not yet flowered will yield a taste that is less bitter.

If you buy dandelion greens that have been cultivated commercially, expect to see red or whitish green stems. The leaves do not last long at all, so store them in the refrigerator inside a plastic container with a piece of paper towel to soak up excess condensation and moisture. You can keep them for as long as four days using this method.

Dandelion greens are among the more bitter greens, so you will want to pair them with a fruit that is especially sweet and flavorful. Some common examples include pineapple, citrus, mango and strawberries.

If you are still new to green smoothies, try a cup or small handful in each serving. As time goes by, you can build this up to four cups.

Radish Greens

You probably would quit green smoothies altogether if you drank one that included blended radishes. However, radish greens are a completely different ballgame. Most of the time, we throw away the radish greens when we are cooking because we do not know the potential of the greens.

When you throw the greens away, you are tossing a great source of iron, magnesium, folate, vitamins A, C and K, and other nutrients as well. In fact, radish greens are much more nutritious than the radishes. Unlike the radish, radish greens are not bitter and they taste much like lettuce. You can mask them with fruit just as easily as you can mask baby spinach.

When you make a smoothie, you'll need a whole radish worth of greens, and you might need to add some more greens in the form of spinach, dandelion or kale. You can get away with as much as two cups of the radish greens and still conceal the flavor with fruit.

When you are choosing radish greens, they are generally attached to radishes. Wash them thoroughly in water so that you eliminate all the debris. Look for leaves that are bright green; avoid any that are yellowing or show any signs of wilting.

10: Principles of a Focused Green Smoothie Diet

Now that you have dozens of recipes and understand the principles behind the green smoothie, here's how a weeklong cleanse works.

When you finish the cleanse, your body will have eliminated many of those toxins that lead to such problems as reduced energy, poor digestion, difficulty sleeping, cravings, bloating, and weight gain. You may think that weight loss is your primary goal, but the other elements of the transformation – brighter and clearer skin, increased energy, better organization, more focus, and better sleep – are just as important to your wellness over the long haul.

For the seven days, you will have three smoothies as your main meals. This means you will be taking in 48 ounces of smoothie every day, 16 ounces at each meal.

However, you should not only eat those smoothies as your sole nutrition. Keep something to snack with you at all times, because your body will rebel against the changes your nutritional regimen is making. If you eat a typical Western diet, you get more than half of your calories from processed carbohydrates, so a green smoothie cleanse is a shock to the system.

What should you have in your snack bag? Cucumbers, tomatoes, celery, apples, melon, berries, and other crunchy vegetables are all permitted. If you want nuts or seeds, you can have a handful a day, but they must be unsalted and raw. Every three or four hours, you should either have a smoothie or a snack to fight off cravings.

During the middle of the day, add a mixed salad to your regimen. The only ingredients of your salad should be raw, fresh vegetables. If you use a dressing, make sure that it has a vinegar base.

You also need a lot of water, about 80 ounces a day. You also have the option of drinking detox tea as the day goes by. You can expect to go through the symptoms of detox during your seven-day cleanse. You'll get headaches, feel cravings and endure fatigue at times. The green smoothies may also give you an energy boost, though, which is a definite plus. The precise reaction that you will have varies from individual to individual.

There are some foods that you must stay away from all week long. These include sugar, milk, meat, beer, cheese, coffee, liquor, sodas (regular and diet), processed or fried foods, and refined carb sources such as donuts, pasta and bread.

Make sure to have some leftover smoothie to leave in the refrigerator overnight. If you commit to drinking some of the extra smoothie if you wake up with a hunger craving, you'll find that it is easier to stay to the plan all week long.

Misery loves company, which means that you will have an easier time completing your cleanse if you have a friend doing it at the same time. If you have someone to keep you accountable, you are much more likely to stay on track with the plan.

You may be wondering whether the detox symptoms can get too severe for the cleanse to continue. Remember that detox is a process of removing wastes and toxins from your body. If you use a green that has a lot of chlorophyll, that chemical actually blends with toxins and pulls them out of your body. This process involves a significant amount of shock to your system, so do not be surprised if this cleanse involves some discomfort for you.

In addition to the headaches and fatigue I mentioned above, there are some other responses that your body may have with the green smoothie cleanse. You may notice a thick coating on your tongue, or a metallic taste in your mouth. You might experience some breakouts of acne or a slight rash. In your nose, you may notice that your body is producing excess amounts of mucus. You may also notice some alterations in your digestive system. Symptoms like gas with a particularly foul odor, frequent trips to the bathroom for a bowel movement, bloating and diarrhea all can occur.

Do not worry if these symptoms appear. While they are not pleasant, they are also a sign that your body is eliminating toxins. Green smoothies are an effective way to get these substances out, and they are milder than some of the other types of detox methods. Once the cleanse ends, those symptoms should clear up in a few days as well.

If you are nervous about these symptoms and this will be your first green smoothie cleanse, you have several options. First, start with one green smoothie a day and gradually build up to the full cleanse regimen. This means that the detox will take longer and you will not experience these symptoms as severe as your body will get accustomed to the ingredients in the green smoothies.

You can also start with a lower proportion of greens than the recipes indicate. Having fewer greens in your green smoothie reduces the detox benefit, but it also reduces the digestive symptoms.

Another way to make the symptoms less unpleasant is to make sure that you drink enough water. Also, go to bed earlier than you are accustomed to. Your body will thank you for the additional sleep, and many of the symptoms will go unnoticed while you are off in lullaby land. Before you know it, the seven days will be up.

So what happens once the cleanse is over? Don't run down to your favorite fast food outlet and buy a greasy burger and fries. You might be tempted to after downing all those fruits and vegetables for a week. However, introducing that oily, fatty food to your system will produce a shock that makes your first reaction to a green smoothie seem gentle in comparison. Your body will rebel against the processed fats and carbs in order of burgers and fries because now it is used to the nutrients that comes from smoothies, salads and healthy snacks.

Instead, add proteins back one at a time, using the lean ones like fish and grilled chicken. Make sure to keep vegetables and fruits as the major components on your plate. Over time, you can add other foods back, and there will be a time when that cheeseburger won't send your intestines into revolution. But will you want it then? Or will you be ready for another week of cleansing? For most people who are devoted to their own health, another cleanse is more likely than a return to the drive-through lifestyle.

Conclusion

If you have never tried a green smoothie cleanse before, you are headed to a completely new level of wellness and energy. It can be intimidating to pick up a glass that contains a thick green liquid and drink it down, but the truth is that green smoothies don't taste all that different from pink, orange, red and yellow ones. The main difference is one of nutrition and fiber rather than one of taste.

The green color in these smoothies comes from chlorophyll. You probably learned in middle school that this is the color that helps plants conduct photosynthesis; it is also this color that connects on a molecular level with the toxins in your system and pulls them out, one at a time.

At first, the removal of these toxins will produce a reaction of nausea, fatigue and pain, but as these chemicals leave your body, you will feel better. Think of a series of pipes that are clogged with gunk and goo – those are your intestines operating on the Western diet. With a green smoothie cleanse, you're cleaning your system out, and the energy you feel will become addicting.

The first seven-day cleanse that you go through will show you how radically an alteration in your diet will improve your life on a number of levels. It is the next series of cleanses that you go through that will convince you that healthy eating is the best way to live.